The Clean Eating Cookbook:

Fresh and Healthy Recipes

By

Jerry   daniel

Table of Contents

Introduction

Here's a sample introduction for "The Clean Eating Cookbook: Fresh and

Welcome to "The Clean Eating Cookbook: Fresh and Healthy Recipes." In a world inundated with processed foods and quick-fix meals, the essence of nourishing our bodies with whole, unadulterated ingredients has become more crucial than ever. This cookbook is a celebration of the power and simplicity of clean eating—a lifestyle that revolves around consuming foods in their most natural and unprocessed state.

Understanding Clean Eating

Clean eating isn't a diet; it's a way of life—a conscious decision to fuel our bodies with foods that are as close to their natural form as possible. It's about embracing fresh fruits, vibrant vegetables, whole grains, lean proteins, and healthy fats while minimizing or avoiding processed and refined foods, additives, and excessive sugars and salts.

Why Fresh and Healthy Matter

The significance of fresh and healthy ingredients cannot be overstated. Not only do they offer an abundance of essential nutrients, vitamins, and minerals, but they also contribute to our overall well-being. By choosing foods that are nourishing and unprocessed, we embark on a journey to optimize our health, enhance our energy levels, and promote longevity.

The Benefits of Adopting a Clean Eating Lifestyle

By adopting the principles of clean eating, we can experience a myriad of benefits. From increased energy and improved digestion to better mental clarity and a strengthened immune system, the advantages extend far beyond just the food on our plates. Clean eating isn't about deprivation; it's about embracing a diverse range of delicious and nutritious foods that support our bodies and enhance our quality of life.

In "The Clean Eating Cookbook: Fresh and Healthy Recipes," you'll find a collection of delectable recipes carefully curated to showcase the beauty and flavors of whole foods. Whether you're seeking vibrant breakfast ideas, nourishing lunch options, or satisfying dinners, this cookbook aims to inspire and empower you on your clean eating journey.

"The Clean Eating Cookbook: Fresh and Healthy Recipes" is your gateway to a world of flavorful, nutritious meals that celebrate the essence of clean eating. Within its pages, you can expect an array of recipes curated to align with the principles of clean eating—centered around whole, unprocessed ingredients that nourish the body and support overall well-being.

Diverse and Wholesome Recipes: Anticipate a collection of diverse recipes spanning various meal categories. From energizing breakfasts that kickstart your day to satisfying lunches, wholesome dinners, and delightful snacks and desserts, each recipe is crafted to showcase the delicious possibilities of clean eating.

Emphasis on Freshness: Fresh produce takes the spotlight in these recipes. Expect colorful fruits, vibrant vegetables, whole grains, lean proteins, and healthy fats as the primary components. These ingredients form the foundation of each dish, emphasizing flavor, nutrients, and the joy of eating whole foods.

Nutrient-Dense Creations: Every recipe is designed to provide not only delightful flavors but also an abundance of essential nutrients, vitamins, and minerals. The focus is not just on taste but on enhancing your overall health and vitality through the food you consume.

Balanced and Accessible: Whether you're new to clean eating or a seasoned enthusiast, the cookbook caters to all levels. It offers balanced meal options, practical tips for ingredient sourcing, and cooking techniques that are accessible to anyone keen on embracing a cleaner, healthier lifestyle.

Encouragement and Guidance: Beyond the recipes, the cookbook offers insights, tips, and guidance on adopting and maintaining a sustainable clean eating routine. It aims to empower you with knowledge, encouraging mindful eating practices and providing support on your journey to wellness.

Versatility and Exploration: Get ready to explore a variety of flavors and cuisines.

From comforting classics with a healthy twist to innovative and creative dishes, the cookbook encourages experimentation and empowers you to explore the world of clean eating with confidence.

In essence, "The Clean Eating Cookbook: Fresh and Healthy Recipes" is not just a compilation of recipes; it's a companion on your quest for a healthier lifestyle. It invites you to embrace the joy of cooking with fresh, nourishing ingredients while reaping the rewards of cleaner eating for your body and mind.

Essentials for Your Clean Eating Journey with "The Clean Eating Cookbook: Fresh and Healthy Recipes"

Embarking on a journey toward a cleaner, healthier lifestyle through the pages of "The Clean Eating Cookbook: Fresh and Healthy Recipes" can be an exciting and transformative experience. As you prepare to dive into this culinary adventure, having the right tools and mindset can significantly enhance your journey toward cleaner eating habits.

1. Fresh Produce and Ingredients

The cornerstone of clean eating is incorporating fresh, whole, and unprocessed foods into your meals. Ensure your kitchen is stocked with a variety of colorful fruits, vibrant vegetables, whole grains, lean proteins, and healthy fats. Think seasonal produce for maximum flavor and nutritional value.

2. Quality Cookware and Utensils

Invest in quality cookware and kitchen tools to prepare clean and nutritious meals. Essential items may include a good chef's knife, cutting boards, pots and pans, baking sheets, a blender or food processor, and measuring cups and spoons. Having reliable kitchen equipment can streamline your cooking process.

3. Meal Prep Containers

Meal prepping can simplify clean eating by allowing you to prepare and store healthy meals in advance. Invest in reusable, BPA-free containers in various sizes to portion out meals, snacks, and ingredients for easy access throughout the week.

4. A Positive and Open Mindset

Approach your clean eating journey with a positive and open mindset. Embrace the opportunity to explore new flavors, ingredients, and cooking techniques. Be patient with yourself as you transition to cleaner eating habits and celebrate every small step toward a healthier lifestyle.

5. Knowledge and Education

Take time to educate yourself about the principles of clean eating. Understand the benefits of different food groups, the impact of processed foods on your health, and how to make informed choices when grocery shopping. "The Clean Eating Cookbook: Fresh and Healthy Recipes" can serve as an excellent educational resource.

6. Support and Community

Surround yourself with support and encouragement. Engage with communities, online forums, or social media groups dedicated to clean eating. Sharing experiences, tips, and recipes with others on a similar journey can be motivating and inspiring.

7. Consistency and Balance

Remember that consistency and balance are key to sustainable clean eating. Aim for gradual changes in your eating habits rather than drastic overhauls. Strive for a balanced approach, allowing occasional indulgences while primarily focusing on nourishing your body with wholesome foods.

Final Thoughts

As you prepare to delve into "The Clean Eating Cookbook: Fresh and Healthy Recipes," gather these essentials to support your journey toward cleaner eating habits. Approach this experience with enthusiasm, armed with fresh produce, quality kitchen tools, a positive mindset, and the determination to prioritize your health and well-being.

Let the recipes within the cookbook serve as your guide, empowering you to create flavorful, nutrient-packed meals that support a cleaner and healthier lifestyle.

Chapter 1:

Breakfasts to Kickstart Your Day

Mornings set the tone for the day ahead, and what better way to begin than with a nourishing breakfast? This chapter is dedicated to revitalizing your mornings with nutrient-rich, flavorful breakfast options that fuel your body and mind.

Nutrient-rich Breakfast Bowls

- Acai Berry Bowl: Packed with antioxidants and topped with fresh fruits and nuts.
- Chia Seed Pudding: A creamy, protein-packed delight with various topping options.
- Quinoa Breakfast Bowl: protein-rich and customizable with fruits and seeds.

Fresh Fruit Smoothies and Juices

- Green Goddess Smoothie: A blend of leafy greens, fruits, and superfoods for a nutrient boost.
- Tropical Fruit Smoothie: Bursting with pineapple, mango, and coconut water for a refreshing start.
- Citrusy Sunshine Juice: A zesty mix of oranges, grapefruits, and a hint of ginger for an invigorating drink.

Whole Grain Pancakes and Waffles

- Banana Oat Pancakes: gluten-free and fiber-packed, topped with fresh berries.
- Blueberry Buckwheat Waffles: Nutritious and crispy waffles served with a berry compote.
- Whole Wheat Apple Cinnamon Pancakes: Comforting flavors perfect for a cozy morning.

Each recipe in this section is crafted to provide a balance of essential nutrients, whether you're in the mood for a creamy breakfast bowl, a refreshing smoothie, or a comforting stack of pancakes or waffles. These options aim to elevate your mornings and set a positive tone for the rest of your day.

Chapter 2:

Energizing Lunches

Lunchtime offers a chance to refuel and revitalize your energy levels. This chapter presents a selection of vibrant and nourishing lunch options that will keep you feeling satisfied and energized throughout the day.

Vibrant Salad Creations

- Mediterranean Quinoa Salad: A colorful blend of quinoa, fresh vegetables, and a zesty dressing.
- Kale and Chickpea Power Salad: Packed with protein and nutrients for a hearty lunch.
- Rainbow Veggie Bowl: A vibrant mix of seasonal veggies with a flavorful tahini dressing.

Wholesome Grain and Protein-based Bowls

- Teriyaki Tofu and Brown Rice Bowl: A protein-packed bowl with savory flavors.
- Mexican-inspired Black Bean Quinoa Bowl: Loaded with fiber, protein, and spices for a satisfying meal.
- Grilled Chicken and Veggie Grain Bowl: A balanced combination of grains, lean protein, and colorful veggies.

Nourishing Soups and Stews
- Spicy Lentil Soup ; A comforting bowl packed with protein and spices.
- Roasted Vegetable and Chickpea Stew: Hearty and nutritious, perfect for colder days.
- Tomato Basil Quinoa Soup: A twist on classic tomato soup, enriched with quinoa for added texture and protein.

These lunch options are crafted to provide a balanced combination of nutrients.

incorporating whole grains, lean proteins, and plenty of fresh vegetables. Whether you prefer a hearty salad, a protein-packed bowl, or a comforting soup, these recipes aim to invigorate your midday meal and keep you fueled for the remainder of your day.

Chapter 3:

Wholesome Dinners

Dinner is an opportunity to unwind and nourish yourself with comforting yet nutritious meals. This chapter offers a collection of flavorful and wholesome dinner recipes that celebrate fresh ingredients and vibrant flavors.

Colorful Veggie-Centric Dishes

- Roasted Vegetable Quinoa Bowl: A medley of oven-roasted vegetables served over fluffy quinoa.
- Stuffed Bell Peppers: Filled with a savory mix of grains, beans, and spices.
- Zucchini Noodles with Pesto: A lighter take on pasta, bursting with fresh flavors.

Lean Protein Entrées

- Grilled Salmon with Mango Salsa; A delightful combination of omega-3-rich salmon and tropical fruit salsa.
- Herb-Crusted Chicken Breast: Tetendernd flavorful chicken breasts coated in fresh herbs.
- Tofu Stir-Fry with Vegetables: A colorful and protein-packed vegetarian option.

Flavorful Plant-Based Meals
- Chickpea and Spinach Curry: A comforting and aromatic dish packed with plant-based protein.
- Eggplant and Lentil Moussaka: A hearty, layered casserole with Mediterranean flavors.
- Quinoa Stuffed Portobello Mushrooms: A satisfying and savory vegetarian option.

These dinner recipes showcase the versatility of fresh ingredients, whether it's through vibrant vegetable-centric dishes, flavorful protein-based entrées, or comforting plant-based meals. By incorporating a variety of textures and flavors, these recipes aim to make dinnertime a delightful and wholesome experience.

Chapter 4:

Satisfying Snacks and Sides

Between meals, having satisfying and nutritious snacks or sides can be both delightful and energizing. This chapter introduces a selection of flavorful and wholesome options that can complement your meals or serve as standalone treats.

Nut and Seed Snack Mixes
- Spiced Almonds and Pumpkin Seeds: A crunchy blend with a hint of heat and savory spices.
- Trail Mix with Dried Fruits: A balanced mix of nuts, seeds, and dried fruits for on-the-go snacking.
- Coconut Maple Granola Clusters: Sweet and crunchy clusters perfect for snacking.

Fresh Veggie Dips and Salsas

- Classic Guacamole: cream avocado with fresh lime and cilantro.
- Mango Salsa: A sweet and tangy salsa with ripe mango, tomatoes, and herbs.
- Greek Yogurt Spinach Dip: A healthier take on a creamy classic, packed with spinach and herbs.

Baked Sweet Potato Fries and Other Healthy Sides

- Baked Sweet Potato Fries: Crispy on the outside, tender on the inside, seasoned to perfection.
- Quinoa and Black Bean Stuffed Peppers: A colorful and nutritious side dish or snack option.
- Cucumber Salad with Herbs: Refreshing and light, a perfect accompaniment to any meal.

These snack and side recipes are designed to offer a balance of flavors and textures while providing wholesome alternatives to traditional snack options. Whether you're craving something crunchy, a fresh dip with veggies, or a nutritious side to complement your meal, these recipes aim to satisfy your snacking desires while promoting healthy eating.

Chapter 5:

Sweet and Healthy Treats

Indulging in sweet treats doesn't have to compromise your commitment to healthy eating. This chapter presents a selection of delightful and wholesome dessert options that satisfy your sweet tooth while aligning with a nutritious lifestyle.

Guilt-Free Dessert Options
- Dark Chocolate Avocado Mousse: creamy, rich, and loaded with healthy fats.
- Berry Chia Seed Pudding Parfait: Layers of chia seed pudding and fresh berries for a nutritious delight.
- Banana-Oat Cookies: naturally sweetened and perfect for a guilt-free treat.

Fruit-based Sweets and Frozen Treats
- Mixed Berry Frozen Yogurt Bark: A refreshing and fruity frozen dessert.

- Watermelon Mint Popsicles: Naturally sweet and hydrating popsicles for a hot day.
- Grilled Pineapple with Honey and Cinnamon: A simple yet indulgent dessert with natural sweetness.

Nutrient-Dense Baked Goods

- Carrot Cake Muffins: moist and flavorful, packed with grated carrots and nuts.
- Whole Grain Fruit Crisp: A comforting dessert featuring seasonal fruits and a wholesome crumble topping.
- Almond Flour Brownies: Rich and decadent brownies made with nutritious almond flour.

These dessert recipes offer a healthier twist on classic sweets, utilizing natural sweeteners, fruits, and nutrient-dense ingredients. By incorporating wholesome elements, these treats aim to satisfy cravings without compromising on taste or nutrition.

Chapter 6:

Tips for a Sustainable, Clean Eating Lifestyle

Adopting a clean eating lifestyle isn't just about recipes—it's about fostering sustainable habits that support your journey toward better health. This section offers practical tips and guidance to help you integrate clean eating into your daily routine seamlessly.

Meal Prep and Planning Techniques
- Batch Cooking: Streamline meal prep by cooking large batches and storing portions for the week.
- Weekly Meal Plans: Plan your meals ahead to avoid impulse eating and ensure balanced nutrition.
- Pre-cut and Washed Produce: Prepare fruits and veggies in advance for quick and easy access during the week.

Smart Shopping for Fresh Produce and Ingredients

- Shop Seasonally: Opt for seasonal produce for fresher, more flavorful meals and to support local farmers.
- Read Labels: Learn to decipher food labels to avoid heavily processed or unhealthy ingredients.
- Buy in Bulk: Purchase staple ingredients like grains, legumes, and nuts in bulk for cost-effectiveness.

How to Maintain a Clean Eating Routine

- Moderation, Not Deprivation: Embrace balance and occasional indulgences while staying mindful of portion sizes.
- Stay Hydrated: Drink plenty of water throughout the day to support overall health and digestion.
- Mindful Eating Practices; Slow down, savor each bite, and listen to your body's hunger and fullness cues.

Incorporating Exercise and Well-being

- Regular Physical Activity: Pair clean eating with a consistent exercise routine for holistic well-being.
- Mindfulness and Stress Management: Prioritize mental health through mindfulness, meditation, or stress-relieving activities.

Creating a Supportive Environment
- Share and Learn: Engage with communities, online forums, or groups to share experiences and gather new ideas.
- Involve family and friends: Encourage a supportive environment by involving loved ones in meal planning and preparation.

By implementing these tips and strategies, you can cultivate a sustainable, clean eating lifestyle that goes beyond just what's on your plate. It's about establishing habits that nourish both your body and mind, fostering a healthier and happier you.

Conclusion

Reflecting on Your Clean Eating Journey

As you conclude this culinary exploration through "The Clean Eating Cookbook: Fresh and Healthy Recipes," take a moment to reflect on the journey you've embarked upon toward a healthier, more vibrant lifestyle.

Embracing the Power of Clean Eating

Throughout this book, you've discovered the incredible potential of clean eating—a lifestyle centered on nourishing your body with whole, unprocessed foods. By incorporating these principles into your daily routine, you've not only diversified your palate but also fortified your body with essential nutrients, vitamins, and minerals.

Empowerment Through Wholesome Choices

Every meal, snack, and dessert has been an opportunity to make wholesome choices that fuel your body and mind. Whether it was starting the day with a nutrient-packed breakfast or indulging in a guilt-free dessert, you've witnessed firsthand the impact of these choices on your overall well-being.

Continuing the Journey to Wellness

Remember, clean eating isn't a destination but a journey—a journey marked by mindfulness, balance, and the continuous pursuit of health and vitality. As you step forward, carry with you the knowledge and empowerment gained from this cookbook.

Gratitude and Encouragement

We extend our heartfelt gratitude for your joining us on this culinary voyage. We hope these recipes have brought joy to your kitchen and inspired you to prioritize your health through delicious, nourishing meals.

Stay curious and stay healthy.

As you close this chapter, embrace curiosity in exploring new flavors, ingredients, and cooking techniques. May your dedication to a clean eating lifestyle continue to empower you, supporting a vibrant and thriving life ahead.

www.ingramcontent.com/pod-product-compliance
Lightning Source LLC
Chambersburg PA
CBHW050754250726
48662CB00005B/2214